Strong for Life

Conor O'Shea

Strong for Life

Copyright © 2023 Conor O'Shea
Print Edition

All rights reserved. No part of this book may be used or reproduced by any means, graphic, electronic, or mechanical, including photocopying, recording, taping or by any information storage retrieval system without the prior written permission of the author except in the case of articles and reviews permitted by copyright law.

Dedication

To Dad, for teaching me there's always an alternative and supporting me along the road less travelled.

Table of Contents

Who should read this book?	vii
My Promise to you	xi
Introduction	xv
Plan	1
Mindset	13
Sleep	24
Move	36
Eat	45
Train	63
Integrate	93
8 Week Strong for Life Program	99
Thank You	125
About the Author	127
The Strong for Life Podcast	129

Who should read this book?

Time is your most precious resource so I want to be upfront with you from the beginning. Let me be crystal clear on exactly who I wrote this for so you can decide if *Strong for Life* is the book for you.

I wrote *Strong for Life* for busy professionals who don't have time to figure out the intricacies of training, nutrition and implementation.

They all have one thing in common: they want to build a body they can rely on without wasting hours working out. They aren't aiming to become the top 1% of athletes, bodybuilders or special operators – they just want a body that is strong, lean and pain-free.

They want 20% information that will give them 80% results without sacrificing family or finances along the way.

If you've tried tons of different approaches, but don't seem to be getting anywhere, then this book is for you.

The *Strong for Life* blueprint is *NOT* for the person who is worried about:

- The exact rep ranges to optimise muscular hypertrophy and performance.
- The exact macro and micro nutrient amounts to optimise fat loss.
- How to become the top 1% of their given sport.
- Optimal nutrient timing for performance.

The *Strong for Life* book *IS* for the person who is focused on:

- Time efficiency.
- Speedy results.
- Training approaches with low risk/ high reward.
- A plan that doesn't require a huge amount of training and nutrition experience.

- A plan they can implement and follow long term, not just for 30 days.
- An approach that gives them more energy, confidence and awareness.

So, if all this sounds good to you… please keep reading!

My Promise to you

If you're still with me, I promise not to waste your time. I truly hope this book gives you clarity on how to approach training and nutrition in a way that feels manageable and effective for your busy life.

I've been coaching for over 12 years and I'll do my part by sharing everything I've learned in that time. Not just the theory, but also how to successfully integrate it into your life long term.

In return, I need you to do your part too. Make the commitment to read this book in its entirety and with an open mind. This book will show you the most effective way to:

- Create time in your week to train and eat well.
- Improve your recovery and sleep quality.

- Change your mindset around what you can achieve with your training.
- Get clear on the best nutrition approach for you.
- Follow the best training program to fit your schedule.
- Tie it all together over the next 8 weeks and beyond.

Of course, if you want or need more details, I highly recommend you download **for free** my 8-week strength & mobility program and 4-month meal prep guide. These guides will teach you how to create simple protein meals in minutes to help you stay lean year-round. You can download both here:

www.conorosheafitness.com/workout-plan-and-meal-planner.html

Strong for Life

Introduction

I had just arrived in Brazil, ready to enjoy a two-week holiday and excited to explore the country before me. The reality? I spent the whole trip limping along with terrible foot pain, completely exhausted and drained of energy.

I had pushed myself too hard, didn't listen to my body and didn't give myself time to recover. Pretty bleak right?

In my mid-twenties, I was constantly getting injured. I had chronic plantar fasciitis, excruciating shoulder pain and was always tired.

To make matters worse, at only twenty-five years old, I would be limping back into work as a totally exhausted personal trainer. The thought occurred to me: "If I'm like this at twenty-five, what am I going to be like at thirty-five or forty?"

What person is going to see a personal trainer limping along in the gym and think: "I want to work with him! He can help me! Sign me up!"

Needless to say, it completely destroyed my confidence and filled me with anxiety.

However, it wasn't all my own fault. I remember going to see a well-respected physio who lived locally. The question he had for me was: "Is your foot injury all in your head?" In other words, was I making it up?

He then proceeded to recommend I buy insoles at the tidy sum of four hundred euros. The result? They did little to help my underlying issue.

This book is going to focus on the "big rocks." I will teach you what you should focus on and what you should forget about.

Most importantly, it's going to give you a structure that will build your body and habits from the ground up. You're not going to be expected to start eating chicken and broccoli twice a day and training fourteen hours a week. It's going to meet you where you're at and help you to move towards the goals you want to achieve.

If there's one concept I'd like you to take away from this book, it's the power of *going narrow and deep* with your focus. When you streamline your energy and focus on the big rocks, you get amazing results.

I know how frustrating it can feel when you put in time and effort, but get no return. This is what happens when you go shallow and wide, trying lots of different things, yet not achieving any results.

In my experience and having worked with hundreds of clients over the years, it seems to be the time wasted researching that catches a lot of people out. It's like going down multiple paths, but only a few hundred metres. If you want to get to your destination, you've got to go all the way down one road and forget about everything else.

We're going to focus on the best path for you to follow – the path to become strong, lean and pain-free. We'll also look at consistency – how to continue on that path regardless of what life throws at you. The clients who get the best results with fitness (or anything else) show up regardless of what's going on in life.

I have tried my best to keep this book succinct so you can sit down and finish it all in one sitting. The goal is to have clarity; what to focus on and what to forget. We will be covering the following:

- Plan
- Mindset
- Sleep
- Move
- Eat
- Train
- Integrate

I've written the chapters in terms of priority but feel free to skip to the chapter you feel is most important for you. For example, if you struggle with nutrition and sleep, it's best to focus on these areas first.

Before you continue reading this book, I want you to keep something in mind. If you find yourself thinking: *Yes, but I know this already*, ask yourself:

1) Yes, but am I doing that?
2) Have I mastered it?
3) Do my results prove that I've mastered it?

Information is everywhere but implementation is where I see most people struggle.

Stop consuming and start implementing.

Plan

"Someone's sitting in the shade today because someone planted a tree a long time ago."
– Warren Buffett

Up until a few years ago, I used to keep a rough idea of the tasks I needed to do in my head. Needless to say, I always felt overwhelmed.

After going through a mastermind course in 2019, I was shown how to plan my day effectively. This simple act has transformed how I feel and perform every day. The days that I don't plan are the days that I achieve less.

I look at planning my day as writing a contract with myself about what I will do. When I have a plan, I always end up achieving far more. It's no different than having a program to follow in the gym.

Everything I teach is about keeping things simple and making it easy to integrate into your life.

I recommend planning your week and your day.

The difference between planning and to-do lists is scheduling. When you schedule a task at a certain time, it gives it urgency and accountability.

A 'to-do' list just gets longer. Writing a note that you "need to pick up groceries" is vastly different from scheduling a trip to the supermarket at 5pm on Tuesday.

If you're spending time each day deciding what to eat and when to train, you won't have the bandwidth to keep this up. Decisional fatigue is a real thing.

You'll opt for the easier option like you always have. Set up your training routine like it's an appointment with the doctor. Put it in your calendar at the same time and day each week so you don't have to think about it.

It's important to be proactive, not reactive. When the chaos of the world tries to distract you, planning keeps you focused and on track.

How to plan your week

I like to use a journal to plan my week. A paper journal is better than a laptop or a phone app. You'll avoid internet distractions if you're writing in a journal. Also, it feels good to put your thoughts down on actual paper.

Write down all the MITs (Most Important Tasks) you have for the week on one page.

This can be: training, shopping, cooking, family, work, appointments, hobbies and leisure time. Now on the next page, split it into a grid with Monday to Saturday/Sunday. In each grid, plot which activities you plan on doing each day.

Below is an example from my work week with the tasks I have planned to do over the next week.

Weekly plan

- Workers
- Content
- New article
- Email
- Follow up GYM
- Reply to all clients
- FB group
- PTD
- Programs

Monday
- Email
- Workers

Tuesday
- FB group
- Content

Wednesday
- Follow up GYM
- PTD

Thursday
- New article
- Reply to all clients

Friday
- Programs

Saturday
- Programs

Pro tip: Don't allocate more than 3 MIT's each day. Ideally stick with one. Achieving an MIT will make your day a success.

If you're reading this, I'll assume that being consistent with training and nutrition is the top priority for you so that might be your MIT each day.

How to plan your day

Next, plan your daily routine the night before or in the morning. Set out what you plan on doing every hour the following day. Slot in when you plan completing your MITs. It might look like this:

- 7am – Wake, water, fresh air, shower
- 8am – Breakfast and time with loved ones/ family/ self
- 9am – 12pm – Work
- 12-1pm – Lunch
- 1-5pm – Work
- 5-6pm – Train (MIT)
- 6-9pm – Family, dinner, chores, read/ TV/ hobby/ social
- 10pm – Wind down, brain dump in journal, plan tomorrow
- 11pm – Bed time

What's great about this, is that it can also be used to plan your food. The main area that my clients fall down is food preparation. When they haven't prepared anything healthy to eat, they usually end up getting a takeaway.

Planning what to eat each week, scheduling a food shopping delivery and setting aside a day for batch cooking has a huge impact on long-term changes in body composition.

A simple way of planning your weekly food is this: –

- Have your food delivered on a Sunday.
- Prep & batch-cook on Sunday to cover your meals until Wednesday.
- Do the same on Wednesday.

You'll only have to cook two days a week instead of seven!

Common Challenges

Planning, like any skill, needs to be developed over time. At the beginning, you won't be very good at it, but this is normal so please don't give up. For example, you might start off by over-planning. However, trying to cram too much in will only result in feeling stressed.

I've been there, done that and still get caught in the cycle at times. Sometimes I schedule too many things into my day trying to optimise every moment. The result? I end up feeling overwhelmed.

The best advice for this is: –

- Plan on doing less
- Give yourself enough time to do it

As I noted earlier, 1-3 MIT's is the maximum number of tasks you should commit to each day.

It's helpful to leave some space in your day too. That way, you have an hour or two of free time in case something crops up at the last minute. This is a much better approach.

What's cool about planning is that you'll realise just how much time you actually do have. Furthermore, you'll choose to spend it in areas that are linked to your goals.

If I fall into a Netflix binge and end up watching several episodes, I start to feel like there's not enough hours in the day. That's because I spent three hours watching TV every night! After a week of nightly binges, my house looks like a college dorm!

When that's not the case, I spend those three hours reading, keeping the house in check, spending time with loved ones, cooking and all the other things that make life better.

Why should you start planning?

Planning gives you more control over your time and your life.

You'll realise you have time to fit in the things you want to do. You'll have time to set aside a nice morning for coffee and reading. Or you'll be able to plan a quiet evening where you're feeling calm and ready to sleep.

As part of my nightly planning, I like to do a "brain dump" in my journal too. This is where I make a list of any issues I'm worried about. It could be regarding my job, my physical pain, my relationships or my family.

It's a great idea to start tracking progress. You'll be able to look back in a few years and see the things you were working on. You'll see the challenges and stressors you were having at the time and how your life has evolved since then.

Whatever it is, once it's down on paper, it's much easier to sleep. This practice alone can have an illuminating effect. As a result of journaling, one of my clients realised he was noting the same stresses every night. He ended up making a huge change in his career and his personal life. Prior to journaling, he had been completely unaware of how much these stresses were affecting him.

Journaling helps to increase self-awareness which is key to progressing in all areas of your life. You also start to realise that the small daily behaviours you put into place today, create the person you will be in 1/ 3/ 5 years from now.

> *"All the benefits in life come from compound interest – relationships, money, habits – anything of importance."*
> *– Naval Ravikant*

For the free spirits who don't like being regimented

I get you. You like to decide things on a whim and use your intuition. You don't like being regimented. But the daily and weekly planning is to give you **more** freedom, not less. The important thing is to make it work for you and not cause more stress.

"Discipline equals freedom" is a famous quote from Jocko Willink that I love.

- When you're disciplined to go to bed on time, you wake up on time and feel fresh.
- When you feel fresh, your mood is better and you don't rely on caffeine or sugar to get through the morning.
- When you're not dependent on these things to get you through the morning, you don't hit a sugar-crash in the afternoon.
- When you don't crash from sugar in the afternoon, you don't feel like bingeing in the evening.

- When you don't feel like bingeing on sugar, you feel more energetic to train after work.
- When you go training after work, you feel calmer. As a result, you're less likely to crave alcohol to unwind.
- When you don't need alcohol to switch off, you get a better night's sleep and feel fresher in the morning.

Do you see the pattern here?

Planning is the most important (unsexy) approach to fixing your body's pains and getting the results you've been looking for.

My client Ray found the main benefit of planning was becoming aware of his workouts. When things popped up that were unexpected, he would look at his calendar, see if his workout was going to be missed, and reschedule it to another time in the week.

In the past, these workouts would have been forgotten about. However, planning keeps it in the forefront of the mind. You'll miss fewer workouts and build a consistent malleable routine. The power of these small changes over the course of an entire year is staggering.

Planning tips:

Planning gives you your time back. Chances are you plan your work life but not your home life.

Schedule a time to do your weekly plan (I recommend a Sunday).

Schedule a time that you will plan your day (I would suggest in the evening after dinner or with your morning coffee).

If you use a digital calendar, put this appointment in there too.

Mindset

*"Your body can stand almost anything.
It's your mind that you have
to convince."*

– Andrew Murphy

It's normally the client's mind, not their training, which causes them to fail. A client can be training well, but their perception of how they're doing is skewed. As a result, they tend to quit.

One of the main things I teach my clients is: **Mindset.** I help understand what long-term compliance actually looks like. I teach them about self-compassion and managing their expectations which allows them to build a long-term training practice.

In this section, we will look at:

- Growth and fixed mindset
- The 20-hour rule

- Don't miss twice
- Just step on the mat
- The rule of five
- Embrace the suck
- Self-compassion

Growth and fixed mindset

The first place I start with clients is to teach them about having a growth mindset. This teaching comes from Dr. Carol Dweck's book "Mindset". In her book, she categorises people as having either a growth mindset or a fixed mindset.

If you have a fixed mindset, you believe you're stuck in your current position regardless of what you do. If you have a growth mindset, you believe you'll improve at an activity, given practice and consistency. If your belief is that you'll improve with practice, then you'll train consistently, knowing it will result in a better outcome.

I teach my clients to become more "Growth mindset" orientated. They'll realise that every practice session leads them to improve in the long term.

20-hour rule

The second thing I teach my clients is the "20-hour rule". This idea comes from Josh Kaufman. He explains that it takes about 20 hours to become proficient at any activity. There's another philosophy that it takes 10,000 hours to become an expert. Josh Kaufman argues that it only takes about 20 hours to reach a level of competence. I like to use the example of meditation.

A lot of people know that meditation is good for them, but they just can't get into the habit of doing it. If they look at it through the lens of the 20-hour rule, they'd realise they're just not hitting enough volume.

When I first started meditating, I was only practising for 5-10 minutes several times a week. After a few months, I felt like I was getting nowhere. The fact is, I wasn't practising for long enough.

Let's calculate it: 5-10 minutes x 3-4 times a week = approximately 30 minutes a week. That's only 2 hours a month! I'd need to stick at it for 10 months to hit 20 hours!

A similar thing happened to me earlier this year when trying to learn Spanish. I was attending a 45-minute class with a teacher once a week. After 8 weeks, I dropped off and stopped the classes. On reflection, I hadn't even completed 8 hours of tutoring. I restarted and signed up for 3 classes a week, knowing I would hit the 20-hour mark over the next 8 weeks.

By teaching this rule to my clients, it helps to manage their expectations if they feel results aren't showing quick enough. It's easy to say, "this is taking months and I'm not getting anywhere". However, if you add up the total time you're training, it might just come back to the fact that you need to increase your volume of training. This also applies to new habits you're trying to put in place and how long you've been practising those skills.

Don't miss twice

"Don't miss twice" is a tip that originates from James Clear. It works particularly well with regards to nutrition. There are many times when I notice that a client is doing really well with their diet. Perhaps they have eliminated one the following:

- Dairy
- Wheat
- Refined sugar
- Alcohol

They stick to this every single day religiously. However, if they miss one day, they feel like they've failed miserably. This results in a binge and completely throwing the new behaviour out the window. The problem wasn't that they missed out on one day of routine. The problem was their resultant feeling of failure and the knock-on effect. One day of a *mess up* turned into months of *mess-ups*.

"Don't miss twice" fixes a lot of these patterns. You missed a day? Just get back on the wagon the following day!

"Don't miss twice" also helps you to stop expecting to have long streaks. Streaks are commonly referred to on nutrition and fitness apps. It means that you set yourself a goal each day and you keep practising it so you don't break the streak. It can be a helpful tool, but remember, if you miss one day, you're still in the top 85th percentile.

Just step on the mat

"Just step on the mat" is something Ryan Hurst from GMB Fitness always says and I love it. When resistance is high, when you feel like skipping a day, when you feel tired, it seems as though a 60-minute workout is impossible. However, if you tell yourself: "Just step on the mat," it helps to overcome that resistance. Once you start, you might do just a few minutes of prep. At the end of prep, check in again. If resistance is still high, you might call it a day. However, most of the time, you'll feel better once you've started and you'll end up doing a full session.

The Rule of 5

"The rule of 5" originates from Dan John, a true legend in the fitness industry. He states that out of 5 workouts:

- one will feel good
- one will feel difficult
- three will feel neutral

Knowing this rule helps to manage your expectations. If only 20% of your workouts feel good, then you're probably on track with your training. Clients sometimes feel that they must be doing something wrong if they don't feel awesome about their workouts or if they're not excited to train. The rule of five is really powerful to help them realise that if 20% of workouts feel good, 60% feel neutral and 20% feel difficult, they're actually on track.

Embrace the suck

This final mindset tip is also from GMB fitness:

"Inspiration is best served with a side of realism. The path to greatness starts with sucking and spending an awful lot of time in mediocrity. You have to allow yourself to suck if you ever want to get great."

In other words, if you're practising something you've never done before, you're not going to be good at it. You're actually going to suck. The good news is; everyone goes through this.

I'd like to link this in with the 20-hour rule. If you're willing to suck at something new for 20 hours, you'll get past that initial discomfort. Prior to the 20-hour mark, this would be the point when most people quit. You try something a few times and it feels awful, so you quit. I get it, I do it all the time. Learning Spanish is extremely difficult for me. I suck at it. However, I suck less now than I did a few months ago. Eventually, I won't suck at all. I'll actually sound pretty fluent.

The same applies for handstands, juggling, improving hip mobility, changing nutritional habits and planning your week. Look at everything as a skill that you can improve. Embrace sucking at it in the beginning. Once you lower your expectations, you'll give yourself the space to progress.

Self-compassion

The final step that ties all of this together is self-compassion. When I mess up or when I'm not good at something, I can become my own worst enemy. My inner critic shows up just to let me know how worthless I am.

When I first heard about self-compassion and self-love, it sounded a bit esoteric and fluffy to me. I didn't really resonate with it at all. That was until I read Dr Kristin Neffs' work.

She breaks it down into three parts:

- Self-kindness versus self-judgement
- Common humanity versus isolation
- Mindfulness versus over-identification

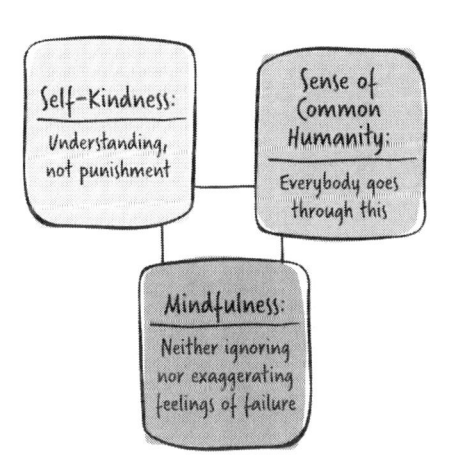

Dr. Kristen Neff: 3 Elements of Self-Compassion

Self-Kindness: Understanding, not punishment

Sense of Common Humanity: Everybody goes through this

Mindfulness: Neither ignoring nor exaggerating feelings of failure

Self-kindness versus self-judgement – Let's say you've just messed up your diet. Instead of judging and criticising yourself, talk to yourself like you'd talk to your best friend. Instead of ridiculing yourself, you'll be more compassionate and remind yourself that it's not a big deal. It's only one day. You've been on track for the rest of the time, so give yourself a break.

Common humanity versus isolation – When I mess up, it can feel like I'm the only person in the world who makes mistakes. Common humanity shows me that the feelings I'm experiencing are also being experienced by thousands, (if not millions), of people right now. Instead of feeling isolated in my struggles, I can remember that this is a common emotion millions of others have experienced.

Mindfulness versus over-identification – When you over-identify with something, you have a belief that it's just part of your character and there's nothing you can do about it. Here's an example: Let's say you order fast food and drink too much alcohol every Friday. You over-identify with this and say: "I can't help myself. I do it every week. I've no self-control."

Having a more mindful approach to this would be to tell yourself:

"Every Friday I get strong cravings to eat fast food and drink alcohol. I also feel really anxious, tired and overwhelmed because I've had such a busy week at work. Maybe if I give myself more time to relax during the week, I won't feel as wound up when it comes to Friday. I won't feel the need to overindulge."

Mindfulness shifts the power back to you. It gives you the ability to figure out why things are happening and awareness to change them. It helps you to take more ownership about making changes in your life. You can apply a growth mindset instead of giving in and believing there's nothing you can do. Over-identification is similar to having a fixed mindset.

Sleep

"Did you know that the supplement industry is twice as big as the entire rest of the fitness and health industries combined? Yeah. Let that sink in."
– Jonathan Goodman

This statistic is crazy, but it shows that people would prefer to take a pill than change their routine. If I offered you a pill and told you it would boost your energy and mood, as well as increase your ability to build muscle and drop body fat, you'd take it, right?

This is what sleep does. It's a super supplement. However, similar to eating vegetables and moving more, this simple advice is difficult to implement consistently.

"Get more sleep" sounds like telling someone to eat less or move more. It's so

simple and obvious, but there are a lot of underlying factors preventing you from better sleep.

Take this quote from Netflix CEO Reed Hastings in 2017:

"You get a show or a movie you're really dying to watch, and you end up staying up late at night, so we actually compete with sleep. And we're winning."

You could get eight hours of sleep or you could watch three more episodes of your favourite new show. Technology is constantly pulling your attention and sleep is what suffers. But it's not just technology, other factors could be loneliness and lack of movement too.

A lot of guys have come into my online program and said they've *"tried everything"* to get results. Sebastian was trying to put on muscle for over six years. When I discussed his lifestyle with him, I could see he was training hard but only getting five or six hours of sleep per night. We first addressed his sleeping patterns, aiming to increase to seven hours and we also focused on his diet. He gained 2 kgs of muscle in two months. Meanwhile, his increased mood and energy made him feel like a new man. We had been aiming to gain 2 kgs in six months, but he achieved it three times quicker than expected! Why? Because he improved his sleep.

When you don't get enough sleep, you wake up tired, craving caffeine and sugar to get you through the day. You start your morning running on a sugar peak and end up crashing like a rollercoaster. You sink into the evening feeling wired which inevitably leads to alcohol consumption to help you wind down. This in turn leads to a vicious cycle of using caffeine to function through the day and alcohol to get to sleep.

I advise my clients to develop three habits which lead to better sleep:

- A 60-minute wind down
- A morning routine
- More movement throughout the day

60-minute wind down

Bedtime routine/ 4 steps to better sleep:

1. Establish a target bedtime and stick to it.
2. Have a comfortable, quiet, dark sleep area.
3. Relax and wind down 30-60 minutes before lights-out.
4. Establish a consistent bed/wake time, even on weekends.

The above step-by-step guide is an example of reverse engineering to get the results you want to achieve. If you're in a cycle of lying in your bed and scrolling on social media until you eventually feel tired enough to fall asleep, it's no surprise if you have sleep issues. That's far too much stimulation in your brain which makes it impossible to shut off. As a result, your circadian rhythm will be completely messed up. Your body still thinks it's the middle of the day!

If you implement the 60-minute wind-down, you'll give your body the chance to calm down so that you're ready to fall asleep when you want to.

Here's what to do:

- Turn off all electronics.
- Write your thoughts down on paper. There are always things rattling around in my mind: "Did I forget…? Tomorrow, I need to do…" etc. Doing a "brain-dump" helps me to get these worries up and out. I recommend buying yourself a journal for this.
- Plan ahead. Set aside anything you might need tomorrow to make the morning easier for you.
- Reading fiction is my favourite final part of this routine. The difference between reading a great book and watching Netflix gives me a vastly different quality of sleep. The problem with Netflix is I end up spending an hour trying to decide what to watch!

Winding Down Suggestions:

- Take a warm bath or shower
- Do some easy stretches
- Listen to audio books or soft music
- Read a fiction book or magazine
- Do a brain dump of your worries/ things to do into a journal
- Write down your wins from the day and what you can improve on next time
- Write tomorrow's plan of how you want the day to go
- Take out clothes for the next morning
- Plan and prep for breakfast

Winding Down Journaling questions:

- What are my MIT(s) tomorrow?
- Do I need to message anyone?
- What 3 wins or awesome things happened today?
- Where can I improve?
- Who did I impact today?

In a perfect world, you'd do this every night. However, the reality is, you might not always have the time. If you can't do it fully, at least try a scaled down version. For example, rather than setting aside 60 minutes, aim to wind down for 10-15 minutes instead. Another concession would be to aim for a 60-minute wind-down from Sunday night through to Thursday night. Then on Friday and Saturday night, you could give it a miss. As long as it fits your lifestyle, that's the key.

10 – 3 – 2 – 1 – 0 for Sleep

To prepare your day for the best possible sleep, I would recommend Craig Ballantyne's **10 – 3 – 2 – 1 – 0 formula:**

- **10** hours before bed – No more caffeine.
- **3** hours before bed – No more food or alcohol.
- **2** hours before bed – No more work.
- **1** hour before bed – No more screen time (turn off all phones, TVs and computers).

- **0** – The number of times you will hit the snooze button in the morning.

Remember, your body adapts to the environment you create for it. So, if your day is nonstop stimulation, your brain is still going to be running overtime when you want to sleep.

Room set-up

The final part of the wind-down is ensuring your room is set up for a good night's sleep. The first step is to make your room as dark as possible. Perhaps your bedroom is exposed to light from the streetlamps outside. If so, it will be much harder to get to sleep so I'd highly recommend you invest in some heavy dark curtains. When I'm travelling and staying in Airbnb's, I use an eye mask if the bedroom isn't dark enough. If I'm really organised, I'll also hang black bin bags or black paper over the windows to ensure a good night's sleep.

Try to reserve your bedroom for sleep purposes only. If you work in your bedroom, your body will associate this room with strenuous brain activity. If you watch

TV in bed, your brain will think it needs to be alert and stimulated. You want your body to associate this room with sleep and relaxation only. If possible, try to use other rooms for work or entertainment.

Morning routine

For the morning routine, I am a fan of Hal Elrod's **SAVERS model**.

SAVERS stands for:

Silence
Affirmations
Visualisation
Exercise
Reading
Scribing

The cool thing about this routine is that it can be completed simply in five minutes. And I do recommend keeping it short. In the past, I would have tried to meditate for forty minutes and then go for a walk and get some exercise. It was great, but the whole thing took about two hours! I needed to get cracking with work and get on with stuff!

So, here's how your morning routine might look for you:

> Wake – 7am – toilet, shower, drink some water
>
> **S** – 7.15 – sit in silence for 1 min, focus on your breath
>
> **AV** – 7.16 – 7.17 – affirmations and visualisation
>
> **E** – 7.17 – 7.18 – Do 60 seconds of squats or walk outside
>
> **R** – 7.18-7.19 – Read a paragraph from an inspirational book
>
> **S** – 7.19-7.20 – Write down 1-3 things you are grateful for

That's it! You can scale these to make it longer, but it's up to you.

Alternatively, you could just pick one of the above and do it for 5 minutes instead. The most important thing to remember is this: if it becomes a huge stressor to you, it's not going to help. So, keep it simple!

Morning Journaling questions:

- What 3 things would make today great? (Controllable activities e.g. workout.)
- What am I grateful for?
- What are my MIT(s)?

Movement

The final part of the sleep equation is to aim to get more movement into your day.

Inability to fall asleep is often due to lack of activity and not feeling tired enough. Coupled with consuming too much caffeine and alcohol, it's easy to get caught in the cycle of feeling too wired at night, using alcohol to sleep, feeling exhausted in the morning and needing caffeine to function.

More movement will help. Aiming to do 10,000 steps each day is a great goal if you struggle with sleep. When you move more during the day, you'll be able to get to sleep quicker and you'll also feel better overall. Your joints won't feel as stiff because they'll be moving more. You'll have less aches and pains. We'll look at this in greater depth in the next chapter on movement.

Timothy was a lifelong early riser and night owl, with understandably poor sleep patterns. When he joined the program, he was averaging five to six hours' sleep per night. After completing the first month of the program, he was already averaging seven hours' sleep each night. He said:

"I'm getting multiple consecutive days of 7+ hours of sleep (and I'm still on that streak). I learned that having a deliberately planned evening wind down period REALLY WORKS!"

Move

"Exercise is optional, movement is essential".
– Unknown

Back in 2013, I sold all my things, packed a bag and went to India. I had been working as a PT for two years, but felt like I needed to travel and see the world. I wasn't happy in the gym I was working at. I felt I wasn't achieving enough or reaching the goals I was capable of. However, I was also petrified of putting myself out there.

India was meant to be a wild adventure. I was hugely excited about the trip, having spent months looking on all the forums and researching my travels.

When I got there, it was anything but exciting.

Sure, it was a massive culture shock, but I spent the first two months teaching voluntarily in Trivandrum, Kerela.

The whole experience was difficult. I taught English without having any plans in place. When I asked my colleagues for teaching advice, they would casually reply: *"Just talk about your life. The kids are very interested in you."*

This worked for about a week. After that, they were bored!

On top of that, I would have to wait after school for a lift back to my accommodation. The waiting time could be anything from ten minutes to three hours. If there's one thing India teaches you, it's patience!

It took me a few weeks to discover that our driver was told to wait until the School Principal had finished his meetings before taking us home. In Indian culture, you don't question a superior. You just wait.

After two months, I'd had enough. I told them I was leaving and I began looking for opportunities to practice yoga instead. Because that's what you do in India – practice yoga, right?

I ended up in a place called Mysore. At the time, I'd never heard of it. If you're not aware, Mysore is a yoga Mecca. It's the birthplace of Ashtanga yoga and it's where the world-renowned "Shala" is. Yoga teachers from all over the world come to Mysore every year to practice.

At that point, I had completed only one month of a Bikram yoga course in Limerick. Needless to say, I was clueless. It's like saying you're into coffee after drinking only Starbucks.

In Mysore, I completed a thirty-day Hatha yoga course, consisting of two hundred hours. It was a big month for me. A lot of light bulbs went off in my head. A lot of realisations. One of which was about the environment I was in.

I had spent most of that month doing yoga and sitting on the ground. I had never sat on the ground before for longer than five minutes. What was alarming to me was how much pain I was in.

My hips and knees were sore all the time. Comparing myself to my classmates and teachers, they seemed to look comfortable. How was that possible? Were they not feeling the agony too? If they were, they were hiding it well!

As the month progressed, my body opened up bit by bit. Sitting on the ground felt easier and as each day went on, I became accustomed to the positions I was spending time in.

By that point, I'd been in India for about three months. It was amazing to observe how the local people moved. Even older people in their seventies and eighties could squat and sit on the ground with ease. Then something clicked. It wasn't that they were doing mobility exercises every week, it was the fact that their environment encouraged movement. They were constantly moving in and out of these positions, so they never lost their mobility.

Look at a preschool child for example. They move with incredible mobility and have perfect squat mechanics. Once that same child has been in school for a number of years, they have lost this capacity.

From the age of 5-25, I wasn't in the habit of spending time sitting on the ground. My body had adapted to the same movements: – going from the bed to the kitchen table, to the car, to the school desk, to the kitchen table, to the couch and back to bed.

Of course, expecting my hips and knees to adapt to sitting on the ground was unreasonable. They had lost that capacity over twenty years ago. If I had maintained this movement throughout my life, it would be effortless.

After four crazy months in India, I moved to Thailand. Going straight to Suan Mok, I began a 10-day meditation retreat. This was another huge challenge for me because it had to be carried out in complete silence. Not only that, but we were also required to sit on the ground for over ten hours each day.

The pain from sitting most of the time was unbearable. It was one of the most challenging, yet also, most rewarding experiences of my life.

Before joining, I remember thinking this would be a cool experience. However, when I woke to the sound of a gong at 4am, panic hit me.

How was I going to get through a full day of sitting from 4.30am to 8pm in complete silence?

Imagine sitting for ten hours each day while your hips and knees feel like they're going to explode! You're trying to meditate whilst at the same time, you're getting eaten alive by mosquitoes. The event took place in an open-air hall where the roof was covered, but that was it. Then at night, you retire to your concrete bed and wooden pillow!

To top it off, people were dropping out of the experience each day. To start with, there were around one hundred people, but approximately ten people left each day. Seeing people give up made the challenge feel even more unbearable!

However, as the days passed, something began to shift. Like most things, I started to get used to it. I let go. I became curious about the pain. I started to separate myself from it. It actually worked.

On the ninth day, we did a 24-hour fast. Food had been the only thing to look forward to. When that was taken off the agenda, there were no crutches left. No external home comforts, nothing left to crave.

Actually, the experience felt freeing. That day, I went into an extremely deep place with my meditation. My pain disappeared and the day flew by.

This experience opened my hips even more. Over the entirety of the ten days, I sat on the ground for over one hundred hours. That was more than in my whole lifetime!

Through these experiences, I started to see how your environment creates you.

I spent another year and a half teaching English and yoga in Khon Kaen, Thailand. I was spending less time sitting in a chair and more time sitting or squatting on the ground. By no surprise, my hips opened more and more. My body felt more supple and mobile. Even my injuries improved.

I followed Ido Portal's 30/30 squat challenge during this time too. The idea is to hold a resting squat for thirty minutes each day for a period of thirty days.

The results shocked me. I had improved my squat much more in that short time than I had in the previous two years put together!

So, the first step towards improving your movement is: –

- Create the right environment
- Practice positions that help to open up your body

For example, if you work from home: –

- Avoid sitting in a chair all day
- Spend some time standing
- Spend some time sitting cross-legged on the floor
- Go for short walks

How can you take advantage of the different ways to add more movement into your day? I like the acronym **OTMs** (Opportunities to move). For example: –

- Can you walk to the local cafe instead of driving?

- Can you take the stairs instead of using the lift?
- Can you jump over the fence instead of walking around it?
- Can you break up your workday with a quick walk around the block?
- Can you spend thirty minutes sitting cross-legged on the floor each day?
- Can you eat your meals sitting cross legged at your coffee table?

These changes won't give you an immediate quick return, but they will compound over the years and give you exponential improvements.

It will also mean you'll end up spending less time and money on physio appointments as you get older!

Eat

"Those who think they have no time for healthy eating will sooner or later have to find time for illness."
– Edward Stanley

There's so much dogma that surrounds nutrition advice. When it comes to food, I want to make this section as simple as possible.

I have followed everything from a plant-based diet to a carnivore diet and everything in between. You don't need to go on either of these extreme diets to get incredible results.

Nutrition is such a charged topic. It can be tough to know what your best option is. For example, it's common to hear <u>both</u> of these statements: –

- *Meat is bad.*

- *Vegetables are poisonous.*

When there's such conflicting views on nutrition, it can get extremely confusing for people.

Clients often ask me: *"What's the best diet?"*

My reply is: *"What would you say if I asked you: What's the best car?"*

I'm guessing you'd respond with: *"The best car for who?"*

A middle-class family in Western Australia will have different transport needs than a single guy in Rome. For the family in WA, an SUV is most likely the best choice, but the 25-year-old guy in Rome? I'm guessing a scooter.

It's the same with nutrition. It depends on the individual.

A carnivore diet is a terrible recommendation for someone who avoids meat for ethical reasons. Alternatively, a vegan diet would be a bad option for someone with IBS.

Josh Hillis has a fantastic way of explaining this by saying: *"Everything is population-dependent."*

A personal example

I have suffered from mouth ulcers my whole life. I was always sensitive to sugar and would be guaranteed ulcers if I ate a lot of refined sugar.

Depending on how clean my diet was or how high my stress levels were, I'd go through phases where my mouth ulcers would flare up.

They got out of hand in 2020. I had moved from Melbourne to Western Australia with my partner at the time. Due to Visa requirements, it was a legal requirement that I didn't work for three months. During those three months, the pandemic hit.

I left my in-person business and had to move my business online, taking an almost 80% cut in salary. I didn't realise it at the time, but I was stressed out of my mind! There was so much uncertainty and my ulcers flared up badly.

I had mouth ulcers for eight months straight. It was horrible. I had problems eating, my energy was completely depleted and the symptoms were similar to depression.

Doctors advised me to take painkillers and use mouthwash. However, this was a Band-Aid, not a cure.

During that time, I tried an autoimmune paleo diet along with a number of other protocols. Nothing helped. Because of the extreme situation I was in, I was willing to try anything.

As a last-ditch attempt, I tried the carnivore diet. Before then, I'd have laughed at the idea, but I was desperate.

After ten days, my ulcers had disappeared.

This was after eight months of trying lots of different diets. Needless to say, the change was staggering.

Ten days, no more ulcers. I need to repeat that sentence because the change was so crazy. It was also life-changing for me. It helped me recover my health. When I get a flare up in the future, I now know what to do.

However, just because it worked for me, that doesn't mean I force my clients to do it.

In fact, I would never recommend a carnivore diet unless you've tried everything else. I certainly wouldn't recommend it to someone who wants to drop body fat.

For another person, I could see how a carnivore diet would cause only negative outcomes such as disordered eating and a feeling of failure.

If you have a low nutritional skill level, you will fail miserably with such a restrictive diet. To better explain, let's look at this through the lens of training.

Let's say two clients come into the gym.

One is similar in fitness to me (let's call him Bob). He's 34, has trained his whole life, is injury-free and can do things like pistol squats, muscle-ups and handstands.

The other is Susan. She's a 56-year-old mother with four children. Susan hasn't engaged in any strenuous physical activity in thirty-five years. She has a stressful corporate management job and suffers from knee pain, hip issues and arthritis in her hands.

Telling both clients to follow the same program would be ridiculous. It might even be dangerous for Susan to follow Bob's program.

Asking Bob to follow Susan's program also wouldn't work. It wouldn't stimulate his body enough and would result in boredom.

So, if you're at a low level of skill and ability with regards to your nutrition, you'll have to learn the basics first. The same with your training.

Doing something like a carnivore diet requires a lot of motivation, but it also requires a lot of nutritional skills. It's an advanced way to eat. For that reason, I would never recommend it to beginners.

The one step I recommend all clients to take universally is to bump up their protein intake.

For ethical reasons, one of my clients had been eating a vegan diet for many years. She was used to eating very little. However, she had also suffered a serious brain injury fifteen years prior which had affected her energy tremendously.

After observing her diet log, it was clear to me that her protein levels were very low.

We increased her plant-based protein intake. After only a few weeks, this was her response:

> *"My energy is the best it's been in years. I can't believe how much better I feel. Thank you!"*

This little tweak changed her life for the better.

How much protein should you eat?

As a simple guide, take your weight number in lbs and convert it to grams to get your recommended amount. I weigh 175 lbs which means I should be aiming for 175 gram of protein each day.

Now to convert that into real food. We can assume most animal proteins (meat, fish, poultry) range somewhere from 20 – 30 grams per 100 pre-cooked. To make it simple, let's call it 20 grams or 20% protein. If I multiply this by 5, I'll get the amount of meat I'm aiming to eat daily to hit my protein.

175 x 5 = 875grams of meat!

If I divide that over 3 meals, that gives me 290 grams of meat per meal. Now that might look like a lot of food because… it is. This is not something you're expected to jump to, tomorrow. You can work on slowly, adding more protein to your diet over the coming months. You can also try to add it to a set number of meals each week. You might aim to hit 290 grams of meat for 5-7 meals each week as a starting point.

Adjust this up or down to fit your body weight.

3 Levers of Nutrition

When you make nutrition work for you, it will dramatically improve your quality of life.

The easiest way to make nutrition work is to follow Dr. Peter Attia's **3-Lever approach:**

3 Levers Nutrition Approach

Restrict what you eat
DR

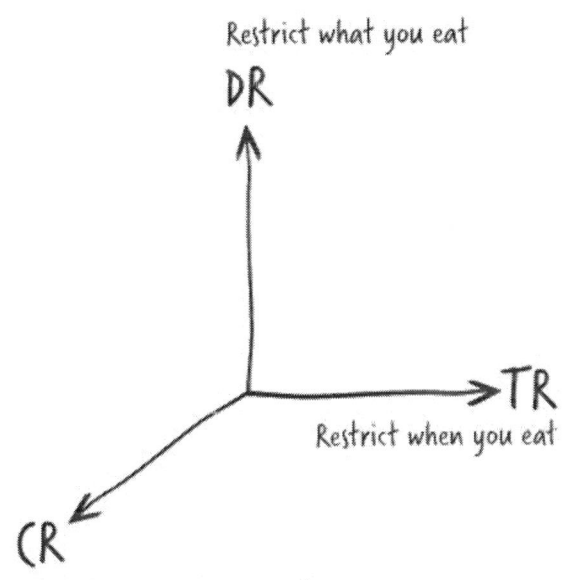

TR
Restrict when you eat

CR
Restrict how much you eat

The 3 levers are: –

1. CR (calorie restriction)
2. DR (dietary restriction)
3. TR (time restriction)

CR – Calorie restriction

Reducing calories – if you track your calories, you might discover that you consume an average of 2,000 calories per day. Drop your calorie intake to 1,800 by weighing your food and keeping track of what you eat. This creates a calorie deficit which will help to drop body fat.

DR – Dietary restriction

Restricting a certain food or macronutrient. For example, you might cut out sugar, dairy, carbs or liquid calories. You'll most likely drop calories as a result of doing this.

TR – Time restriction

Not eating during a certain timeframe. For example, it might be a 24-hour fast once every few weeks. Alternatively, it could be skipping breakfast and only eating between noon and 8pm.

Eating whatever you want, whenever you want and as much as you want is the standard American (Western) diet. After fifty years of research, we can see clearly where that leads you. In case you're not sure, it's: –

- Disease
- Obesity

- Chronic health issues

The goal is simple:

- Always pull one lever
- Sometimes pull two
- Occasionally pull all three

That's it. That's the most effective (non-dogmatic) approach I've ever encountered.

So how might this look? Here's an example of how I eat: –

- I almost always use **TR (time restriction)**. I generally skip my breakfast and eat two meals a day.
- **DR (dietary restriction)** I eat mostly meat and vegetables (a paleo style diet). I also cut out dairy from time to time.
- **CR, TR & DR –** Once or twice a year, I'll do a 2-3 day fast, consuming only water or bone broth. **(Pulling all 3 levers).** *(I only recommend pulling all 3 levers if you have built a good foundation of nutritional compliance).

This works well for me. Someone else might decide to cut out dairy or sugar and focus on DR (dietary restriction). You might prefer to focus on CR (calorie restriction). And that is why it is such an effective system. You can choose what works best for you at this period of your life.

You can pull whichever lever you feel is going to work well for your lifestyle, but make sure you're pulling at least one!

What do I eat?

Now that you are clear on the 3 levers, let's make things clear about what to eat.

Here's a simple framework to think about:

1. Did it have eyes? (Meat, fish, poultry)
2. Did it come out of the ground? (Plants)
3. Did it come out of a tree? (Fruit)

ns For Nutrition Clarity

Did it have eyes? (meat, fish poultry)

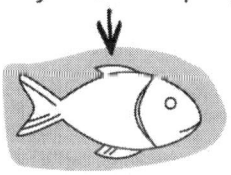

Did it come from a tree?

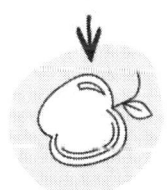

Did it come from the ground?

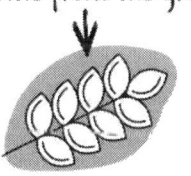

If you can answer yes to any of these questions, you are eating a food that will be beneficial to your health. If it was made in a lab in the past 30 years and has more than five ingredients, chances are, it's not the best option.

Below is an example of what you're aiming your plate to look like most of the time. I recommend aiming for 80-90% of your meals to be made up of minimally processed food cooked at home.

Then you have 10-20% of your meals to play around with each week. If fat loss is the primary focus, you may need to stick to 90% of your meals. If you struggle with guilt when you eat "bad" food, I explain in the next section how to use value-based decisions when choosing food options.

What your plate should look like

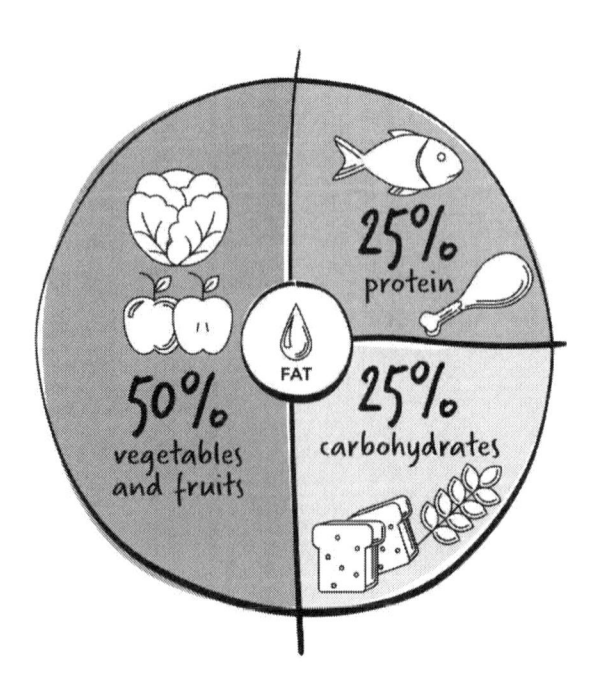

Getting away from black and white rules with value-based decision making

When you begin to use value-based decisions, you'll be able to stop looking at food in a black and white manner. You'll start to enjoy food guilt-free. By using the above-named approach, you'll be able to make better choices around how you use food. You'll stop seeing foods as either good or bad. Josh Hillis led the way in the fitness industry with this approach.

Here are some examples of value-based decision making that I like to share with my clients:

> **Situation 1:** After a stressful week of work, you reach for a bag of chips to shut off your emotions.
>
> **Situation 2:** After a busy week, you decide to connect with a loved one and enjoy a bag of chips together, discussing how your week went.

In the second example, you are actively choosing to enjoy the chips with a loved one. You're not using the chips to bury your emotions.

Even though the food or drink you are having is exactly the same, the motivation behind consuming it is completely different.

One is to escape; the other is to connect.

If your values are around connection, there shouldn't be guilt attached.

In the past, the trap I've found myself in is feeling bad if I use food to avoid emotions. However, I feel equally bad or feel like I'm doing something *wrong* if I actively decide to have dessert with a loved one.

Value based decisions have enabled me to break free of this strange guilt cycle and allow myself to enjoy the foods I have actively chosen to eat. It also helps me to make better decisions around what to do if I feel drawn towards using food to shut off my emotions.

HALT!

Another useful tip for making decisions around food is using the **HALT** acronym.

This stands for:

Hungry

Angry

Lonely

Tired

HALT originated from the addiction recovery world. It is used with addicts to warn them when they are at a "high risk" emotional state and are therefore susceptible to using drugs.

It's a useful acronym to remember if you are experiencing a lot of food cravings. When I feel a strong desire to eat junk food or drink alcohol, I check in with myself and simply ask: Am I hungry, angry, lonely or tired?

Sometimes just acknowledging that I am feeling a specific emotion and sitting with it, is enough to allow these cravings to pass.

Other times, it might mean that I need to address the various issues:

Hungry – I need to prepare a substantial healthy meal.

Angry – I need to work through some emotions.

Lonely – I need to reach out and talk to a friend.
Tired – I need to slow down and get some rest.

Train

"We do not stop exercising because we grow old – we grow old because we stop exercising".
– Dr. Kenneth Cooper

After coaching clients for over a decade, I've noticed that training is rarely just about looking good. There are many other factors at play. Sure, having a 6-pack or a defined chest is aspirational, but I don't think you'd want that at the expense of always having shoulder and back pain, right?

In this section, I'll show you the work I do with my clients, so you can get amazing results too.

I focus on 3 main areas:

1. Improving strength, mobility and motor control to achieve higher levels of movements and skills

2. Injury rehab, postural restoration – offsetting environmental issues
3. Aesthetics – looking good

These three areas all complement each other. Pursuing more strength, mobility and control helps with injury resilience which in turn results in looking better. If I'm getting stronger, doing more advanced movements and staying injury free, my body will look better too.

When you chase aesthetics at the expense of everything else, there doesn't tend to be as much longevity with the training approach.

Why use a skill-based approach?

Using a skill-based approach (ladder of progression) with clients has also helped them improve their training consistently. In the past, I struggled to keep clients engaged in their training when I was using the stock strength training and progressive overload.

"Okay Jack, last week we did 50kgs in the squat, this week we are doing 52.5kg!"

This type of training bored both me and my clients. When we set goals around skills, my job was to deconstruct the movement to a level that was accessible to them. They were then able to see how they were working toward that skill. This instilled a lot of excitement in their training and ability.

Showing a client that their push-up off the knees is leading towards a ring dip or muscle up is pretty exciting. I also use this approach with clients to rehab injuries. We rehab an area and then work towards a skill that's going to be extremely demanding on this area.

When a client has a shoulder injury, I'll help them rehab the area and then help them work towards something like a muscle up. The reason for this approach is twofold. It leads to massive confidence around their now rehabbed area and it also helps them to work through the boring periods of rehab knowing the direction we are taking things.

A lot of exercise rehab has low compliance because clients become bored out of their minds. They end up doing the same banded rotator cuff movements without any road map or plan of where things are going.

My client Matt is a perfect example of this. He went from chronic shoulder and elbow pain for over four years to feeling bulletproof. He can now do ring muscle up variations which are extremely demanding on the elbows and shoulders.

Physical Autonomy

I first heard the term "physical autonomy" during the GMB apprenticeship. Since then, it's a term I always use with clients and it seems to resonate with them a lot.

Physical autonomy means: your training supports the body you want to have, for all the things that are important to you.

For one person, that might mean having the hip mobility to play with their kids on the ground and the shoulder stability to play on the monkey bars at the park.

For someone else, that might mean having the upper back strength to work 8-10 hours a day without getting chronic shoulder and neck pain.

For me, it means having the physical strength to work a 12-hour day (if needed). To be able to hike Mount Teide in Tenerife, to go Freediving in Malta, to carry a 20kg suitcase up six flights of stairs, to have strong feet to dance Salsa, to have the strength and mobility to do handstands and muscle ups for fun.

I spent far too many years living with a body that was always holding me back and worrying about it letting me down. The most important thing to understand about your body is that any issues you have are treatable. However, you need to start training for the things you want to be able to do.

How to decide what to put in your program

There are unlimited ways to design a training program. Every coach has their own style of programming. In this section I'm going to explain how I design fitness programs. I'll explain how I lay them out and what exercises I use. I'll also show you how to set up your own program depending on how frequently you train.

An important part of designing a program is to create structural balance in the body.

The program should help you to:

- strengthen weak body parts.
- increase the range of stiff joints.
- bring more balance to the front and back of the body.

To better understand programming, here are the four areas to focus on:

- Programming framework
- Movement patterns
- Exercise selection
- Training frequency

5 P's programming overview

The 5 P's programming is the main framework I use. It originated from my friends at GMB Fitness and I love it. My clients do too.

This is what it involves:

Prep = your warm-up

Practice = the main theme of the workout or skill you're working on.

Play = working on lower-level movements that are linked to your theme

Push – your standard strength and conditioning movements you're confident with

Ponder = reflection on your session along with stretches linked to your restrictions.

What movements should you do?

In training, we use certain movement patterns and body parts. To keep things simple, here are the main movement patterns we'll focus on:

- Squat
- Hinge
- Upper push – horizontal
- Upper push – vertical
- Upper pull – horizontal
- Upper pull – vertical
- Core, ground movements

We can also use accessory movements for the ankles, lower legs, hips, elbows, wrists and shoulders.

Dan John first popularised this and it's a simple way to audit your training program. A lot of guys tend to focus on beach muscles like chest and arms, neglecting their back and legs.

A quick scan of these patterns helps you to see where your current training approach may be lacking. If you look at the above list and see your gym program has mostly upper pushing and core work, it's obvious you need to add in the squat, hinge and pulling movements to bring more balance to your program.

Understanding tonic & phasic muscles

In the late 60's, Czech neurologist and physiotherapist, Dr. Vladimir Janda, found that certain muscles get tighter whilst others get weaker.

Examples of tonic muscles (muscles which get tighter):

- Pecs (chest)
- Biceps

- Hip flexors
- Piriformis
- Hamstrings

Phasic muscle examples (muscles which get weaker):

- Rhomboids
- Triceps
- Glutes
- Deltoids
- Abs

A simple programming rule is to strengthen the back of the body and stretch the front of the body. This will help to tighten the phasic muscles and lengthen the tonic muscles. There are still tonic muscles along the posterior chain (hamstrings) and phasic muscles in the anterior chain (abs). However, this programming rule can help to fix a lot of issues for clients, especially when you consider how most of us spend our day – hunched over a laptop, phone or steering wheel. This causes the muscles in the front of the body (chest, hip flexors) to tighten and the muscles in the backside (back, glutes) to weaken and lengthen.

These postural limitations are called upper and lower crossed syndrome. In the diagram below you can see how weakness and tightness impacts the upper and lower body.

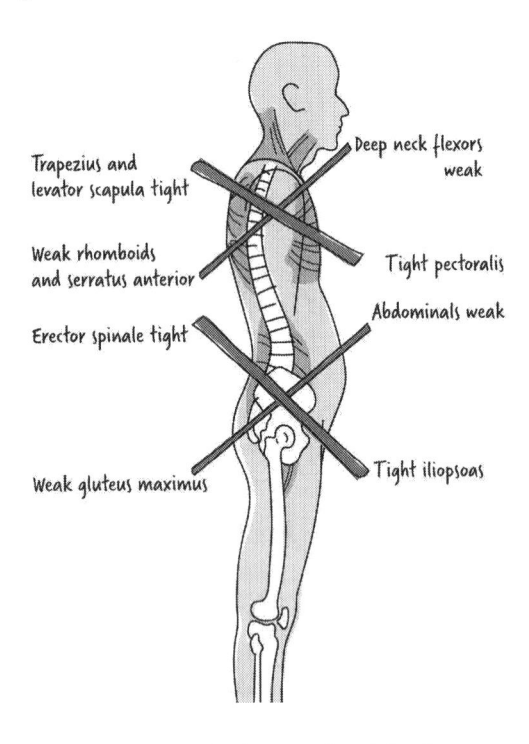

Trapezius and levator scapula tight

Deep neck flexors weak

Weak rhomboids and serratus anterior

Tight pectoralis

Abdominals weak

Erector spinale tight

Weak gluteus maximus

Tight iliopsoas

This diagram helps to highlight many of the issues people find when they start training. When they arrive at the gym as newcomers, their chest/ hip flexors (tonic) are extremely tight, while their upper back and glutes (phasic) are very weak. Starting off their training with gusto, they hit the bench and do curls and leg extensions. Meanwhile, they skip glute work and upper back work. Unfortunately, this causes even more tightness throughout the chest and hip flexors, which often leads to shoulder, hip and lower back issues.

What exercises should I do?

Examples:

- Squat
  Bodyweight squat, Goblet squat, back squat, front squat.
- Single leg squat
  Lunge, reverse step up, split squat, Bulgarian split squat, pistol squat.
- Hinge
  Dowel hinge, DB RDL, Deadlift, kettlebell swing, Snatch grip deadlift, Deficit deadlift, Snatch grip deficit deadlift.

- Single leg hinge
  Back scales, Single leg deadlift, Shrimp squat
- Upper push
  Horizontal – Push up, Ring push-up, dips, ring dips.
  Vertical – Inverted press, overhead press, handstand, handstand push-up.
- Upper pull
  Horizontal – Ring row, bent over row, archer ring row, front lever tuck, front lever.
  Vertical – scapular pull-ups, chin up, muscle-up, archer chin-up, one arm chin up,
- Core/ groundwork
  Plank, dead bug, hollow body hold
  Bear, frogger, monkey
- Accessory movements
  Shoulders – external rotation, trap 3
  Elbows – biceps, triceps
  Wrists – flexion, extension
  Hips – glute medius activation

Ankles – tibialis raise, calf raises

How to choose your movements?

Pursuing skill work is like taking steps up a ladder. With each step, the movement becomes more complex and challenging. Skill training reinforces the importance of good form and technique.

If you rush up one of the steps of the ladder, you won't be able to progress to the next step. Therefore, it keeps you consistent with your progress.

For each of the movement patterns above, imagine they are separate ladders. As you go up the ladder, the movements become more challenging. If you're unsure what level you're at, I recommend starting on the first step.

Horizontal Push skill progression ladder

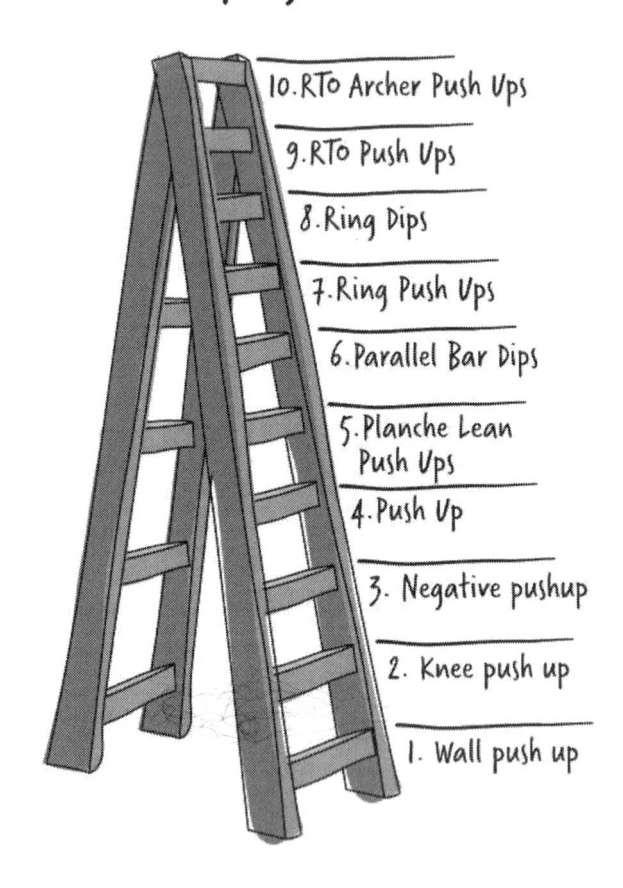

10. RTO Archer Push Ups
9. RTO Push Ups
8. Ring Dips
7. Ring Push Ups
6. Parallel Bar Dips
5. Planche Lean Push Ups
4. Push Up
3. Negative pushup
2. Knee push up
1. Wall push up

Training frequency:

The normal frequency of training options which I encourage my clients to do is:

- 2/ 3/ 4 days per week

Depending on frequency, I recommend you split your training days as follows:

<u>For 2 days a week</u>, I recommend two full body days.

I like to use an 'X split' for this style:

Day 1 – you focus on upper pulling and lower squat patterns.

Day 2 – you focus on upper push and lower hinge patterns.

The reason I like the X split is that it organises your training with movements that don't compete with each other. For example, a chin-up doesn't fatigue any of the movements that the squat uses. They work as a nice pairing instead of chin-ups and deadlifts which tax both the grip and back muscles.

Example 2 day/week workouts

Days of week example: Tuesday & Thursday

Day 1
Prep – Full body warm up

Practice – Chin ups (vertical pull), ATG split squat (single leg squat)

Play – Frogger (squat, ground movement)

Push – Ring row (horizontal pull), goblet squat (squat), dead bug (core)

Ponder – Lunge A (hips), dowel shoulder mobility (shoulders)

This session hits everything from the squat and pulling patterns. There's a combination of single leg and normal squatting, horizontal and vertical pulling and core and locomotion.

Day 2

Prep – Full body warm up

Practice – Bear crawl (vertical press), Single leg RDL (single leg hinge)

Play – Crab (core, groundwork)

Push – Push up (horizontal press), DB RDL (hinge), Superman (posterior core).

Ponder – Pigeon (hip), posterior shoulder opener (shoulder).

This routine hits the hinge and single leg hinge, posterior core and vertical and horizontal pressing. The bear is a safe vertical pressing option. I tend to avoid vertical pressing movements like inverted press or shoulder press initially with clients because it's a "higher risk" movement for the shoulders. Most clients don't have adequate shoulder mobility to execute it safely in the first 3-6 months of training.

For the 3-day split, I recommend spending two days on the upper body and one day on the lower body. With this split, I would focus on an upper pushing day and an upper pulling day. The lower body day would cover squats and hinges.

> 3 day split: Upper pull/ Lower squat/ hinge/ Upper push
>
> Days of week example: Monday, Wednesday, Friday.

Day 1 (upper pull)

Prep – Full body warm up

Practice – Chin ups (vertical pull)

Play – 3-point bridge (core, ground movement)

Push – Ring row (horizontal pull), dead bug (core), bent over T-raises (horizontal pull)

Ponder – Posterior shoulder opener (shoulder), dowel shoulder mobility (shoulder)

Day 2 (lower squat/ hinge)

Prep – Full body warm up

Practice – Goblet Squat (squat)

Play – Frogger (squat, groundwork)

Push – ATG split (single leg squat), DB RDL (hinge), Superman (posterior core)

Ponder – Pigeon (hip), Lunge A (hip)

Day 3 (upper push)

Prep – Full body warm up

Practice – Ring Dip (vertical push)

Play – Bear (vertical push, ground based)

Push – Push up (horizontal push), hollow body hold (core), ring top position (vertical push)

Ponder – Pigeon (hip), posterior shoulder opener (shoulder)

For the 4-day split, I recommend dividing it up as follows:

> Upper push/ Lower hinge/ Upper pull/ Lower squat
>
> Days of week example: Monday, Tuesday, Thursday, Friday

I've organised the days so you are getting maximum recovery. The upper push day is not causing any fatigue to the lower hinge day. You then have a full day between the hinge day and pull day. The pull and squat day are not competing either. In my experience this allows better recovery and lower injury risk.

Example as follows:

Day 1 (upper push)

Prep – Full body warm up

Practice – Ring Dip

Play – Bear

Push – Push up, hollow body hold, ring top position

Ponder – Pigeon, posterior shoulder opener

Day 2 (hinge)

Prep – Full body warm up

Practice – Deadlift

Play – Crab

Push – Reverse step up, Single leg RDL, side plank

Ponder – Pigeon, Lunge A

Day 3 (upper pull)

Prep – Full body warm up

Practice – Chin ups

Play – 3-point bridge

Push – Ring row, dead bug, bent over T-raises

Ponder – Posterior shoulder opener, dowel shoulder mobility

Day 4 (squat)

Prep – Full body warm up

Practice – Squat

Play – Frogger

Push – ATG split, DB RDL, Superman

Ponder – Pigeon, Lunge A

How do I know what split is best for me?

If you are a beginner (who has been training for less than one year) stick to a 2-day split. When starting out, you need to keep repeating the basics, so 2 days per week is going to help you here.

It's also much less overwhelming to learn two days of movements instead of four. If you want to train more frequently, just repeat the days. If you want to train four days a week, repeat each day twice.

Weekly outline (2 days/week example)

Day 1 – Day off

Day 2 – workout 1

Day 3 – day off

Day 4 – workout 2

Day 5 – day off

Day 6 – day off

Day 7 – day off

Weekly outline (3 days/week example)

Day 1 – workout 1

Day 2 – day off

Day 3 – workout 2

Day 4 – day off

Day 5 – workout 1

Day 6 – day off

Day 7 – day off

Weekly outline (4 days/week example)

Day 1 – workout 1

Day 2 – workout 2

Day 3 – day off

Day 4 – workout 1

Day 5 – workout 2

Day 6 – day off

Day 7 – day off

For those of you who have been training longer than a year, it would be advantageous to follow a **3-day workout plan**. This would give you variety and allow you to cover more movements and skills. You can add more days and just repeat the workouts.

Week (3 days/week example)

Day 1 – workout 1

Day 2 – day off

Day 3 – workout 2

Day 4 – day off

Day 5 – workout 3

Day 6 – day off

Day 7 – day off

Weekly outline (4 days/week example)

Day 1 – workout 1

Day 2 – workout 2

Day 3 – day off

Day 4 – workout 3

Day 5 – workout 1

Day 6 – day off

Day 7 – day off

A **4-day split** is generally for someone closer to the intermediate level. They've been training consistently for more than two years. They don't struggle to show up for training four days a week. This is how I train personally. For the majority of people I work with, this is too much and that's totally cool.

I will always train four days every single week. It's part of my week. Some weeks I'll train 5-6 days, but I am always able to show up four times. This also gives me more time to work on specific skills and body parts.

Having a whole day to focus on upper body pressing allows me to spend time doing handstand push-up variations. In a 45-60 minute session, I can also fit in other upper body pressing movements.

If I was trying to do upper body and lower body movements on the same day, it would take over 90 minutes which is too long for me.

If you want to train more than 4 days a week, you can just cycle through the workouts again. So, your week will look like this:

Weekly outline (4 days/week)

Day 1 – workout 1

Day 2 – workout 2

Day 3 – day off

Day 4 – workout 3

Day 5 – workout 4

Day 6 – day off

Day 7 – day off

Weekly outline (5 days/week example)

Day 1 – workout 1

Day 2 – workout 2

Day 3 – workout 3

Day 4 – day off

Day 5 – workout 4

Day 6 – workout 1

Day 7 – day off

Weekly outline (6 days/week example)

Day 1 – workout 1

Day 2 – workout 2

Day 3 – workout 3

Day 4 – workout 4

Day 5 – workout 1

Day 6 – workout 2

Day 7 – day off

A word of caution with your training program

"The coach who trains himself has an idiot for a client."

– Dan John

If possible, I'd strongly recommend you get help designing your program as it's extremely difficult to write your own.

When I write my own programs, I either put in too many things, or I avoid the areas I should be prioritising. That's why I've had my programs written for me by other coaches for over six years.

These programs don't need to be custom built; you can follow a program like GMB's Elements or Integral strength. However, please follow a program written by someone other than you!

How to know how hard you should push yourself?

When you train, I recommend avoiding "training to failure". Even though there are lots of people on the internet telling you to train to failure in order to maximise muscle growth, I disagree.

Instead focus on autoregulation. Below is a graph from GMB Fitness that shows the power of autoregulation. Autoregulation means you adjust things during the workout depending on how you're feeling. So, if your program says 10 reps, you don't hit the 10 reps at all costs. You might do 5 or 6 because you are tired that day.

This becomes helpful for clients who tend to skip working out on the days they don't feel good. When you understand autoregulation, you can always train, just at a lower intensity. You can also apply autoregulation to your habits. I use the term *scaling* habits in the book which is the same as autoregulation.

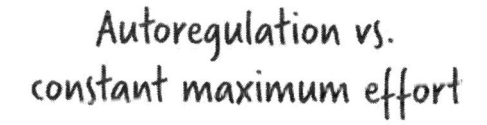

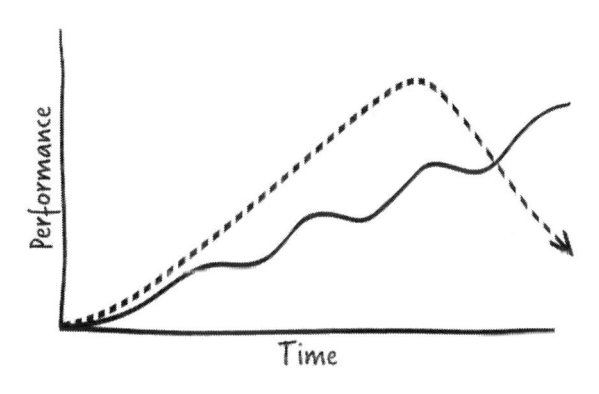

Autoregulation vs. constant maximum effort

----▶ Constant Max Effort
Steep progress often leads to steep declines.

───▶ Autoregulation
Steady progress helps you maintain a high level of performance over time.

More reasons why you shouldn't train to failure

Training to failure increases the risk of injury and you will constantly feel sore. This book is not about teaching you how to become the best athlete or most muscular. It's about teaching you how to create a movement and nutrition lifestyle that makes you feel better overall. You will gain plenty of muscle following the steps I've gone through.

As a rule, I recommend keeping 2 reps in reserve (RIR) when you train or at an RPE of between 7 and 8/10. For example, if you do a set of 8 chin-ups, you could have done 10, but you stop 2 reps before failure. I'll explain below why I prefer this method.

Using the chin-up example, if you go to failure on the first set, here's what the reps will look like (as an example).

Set 1 – 10 reps (failure)
Set 2 – 6 reps (failure)
Set 3 – 4 reps (failure)
Set 4 – 3 reps (failure)
Set 5 – 2 reps (failure)

Total reps = 25

Form was poor and it takes you 3-4 days to recover. There's also a chance that you start aggravating your rotator cuff following this style of training for a few weeks.

In the second example, I'm going to train with 2 RIR.

Set 1 – 8 reps
Set 2 – 8 reps
Set 3 – 7 reps
Set 4 – 7 reps
Set 5 – 6 reps
Total reps = 36

In the second example, you're increasing the volume of reps, yet you'll have better form and be able to train more frequently. Over the course of a year, that's a lot of extra reps which is going to result in much better results

If you want to train to failure, go ahead. However, "going to failure" in each session will most likely cause injury. It will also result in a lack of training consistency due to muscle soreness.

Below is an example of the RPE table that you can also use to better understand how intensely you can train.

RPE Scale
Rating of Perceived Exertion Scale

10	Could not do more repetitions or weight
9.5	Could not do more repetitions, could do slightly more weight
9	Could do 1 more repetition
8.5	Could do 1 more repetitions, possibly 2 more repetitions
8	Could do 2 more repetitions
7.5	Could do 2 more, possibly 3 more repetitions
7	Could do 3 more repetitions
5-6	Could do 4 to 6 more repetitions
1-4	Very light effort

Integrate

"Step 1: Write this phrase on a small piece of paper: I change best by feeling good, not by feeling bad."
– B.J. Fogg, Tiny Habits: The Small Changes That Change Everything

Much of the messaging in the fitness industry is around suffering and restriction. The workouts should be brutal and the diets should be extreme. That's how you get results, right?

Some of the most popular fitness franchises have intense unsustainable workouts. They are novel and sexy, but the workouts are not repeatable. You can't train like that long term.

To integrate fitness and nutrition into your life, it needs to be easy. There's a well-known saying in the business world: *"Under promise, over deliver"*. That's exactly what you need to do with your commitment to training and nutrition. Below is an image from James Clear which really hits home on where people fail with setting the bar to high habits.

"So easy, You can't say no"

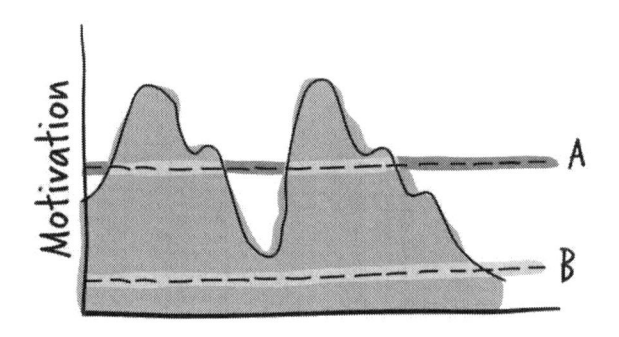

A - Hard, Inconsistent habit

B - Easy, Consistent habit

The push back I get from this with clients is that the habit is too easy and insignificant. But that's the magic of under-committing. You can only get results through consistency and consistency is impossible if the commitment is too hard.

When these same clients see the progress they've made 9 months down the line they're baffled. They get way better results with much lower intensity. The difference is that they never stop.

It works the same as compound interest. If you take all your money out of the market every 3-6 months, you never avail of the magic of compound interest. Your health and habits are the same.

Scaling Habits (Adjust the dial)

In order to succeed in the long term, I teach my clients how to scale their workouts and their habits. In the same way that you can adjust a temperature dial, you can do the same with your habits.

Let's imagine that your overall ability on a dial goes from 1 – 10. For me, reaching a "7" on the dial would be doing 4 workouts a week, along with lots of movement, such as walking or hiking.

However, I can also scale that down to a "3" on the weeks that I'm very busy with work. Reaching a "3" on my dial might equate to a 10-minute workout beside my bed each morning.

The better you get at scaling your habits and workouts, the easier it will become to implement this as a long-term approach. It will also get you past the *"pause button mentality"*.

The "pause button mentality" is when you pause your healthy habits because life has become too busy. When things settle down, you restart your healthy habits. Of course, this results in you pressing pause for six months every year! Scaling your habits allows you to continue working on your routine regardless of how busy you become.

Movement Dial

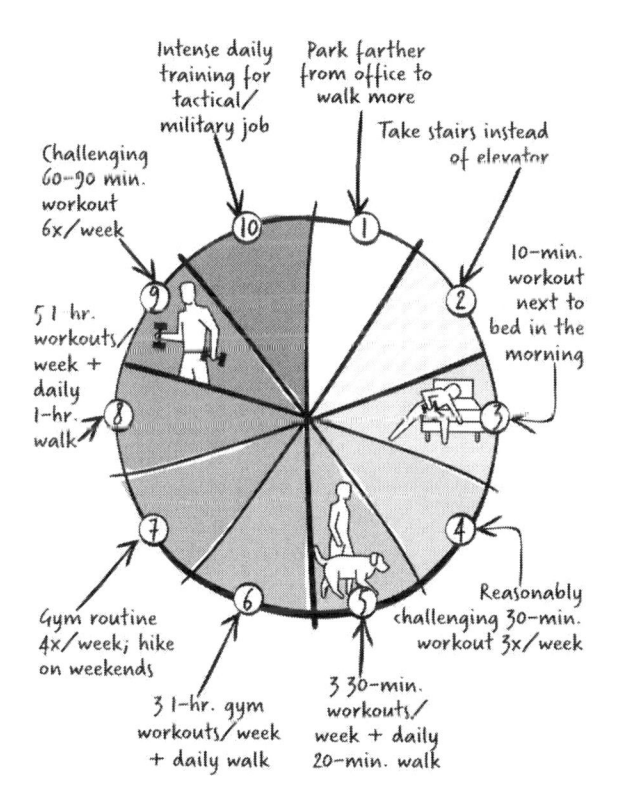

- 1: Park farther from office to walk more
- 2: Take stairs instead of elevator
- 3: 10-min. workout next to bed in the morning
- 4: Reasonably challenging 30-min. workout 3x/week
- 5: 3 30-min. workouts/week + daily 20-min. walk
- 6: 3 1-hr. gym workouts/week + daily walk
- 7: Gym routine 4x/week; hike on weekends
- 8: 5 1 hr. workouts/week + daily 1-hr. walk
- 9: Challenging 60-90 min. workout 6x/week
- 10: Intense daily training for tactical/military job

How to track habits

At this point, I've tried every habit tracking app and system. Simplicity always wins. I love how James Clear tracks habits in a notebook. Tracking is essential for you to stay on track (pun intended). It also gives you accountability. The biggest issue I have with new habits is forgetting to practise them.

Therefore, I've found the easiest way to track habits is to write what I'm working on at the back of my journal, along with the date. I simply tick it off each day that I'm training. I add this to my daily planning so it's streamlined. If I miss a day or two, I just add it in when I next review my planning.

Below is a simple sketch to show how you can do it too. You can also use a spreadsheet but personally I prefer to do this by hand in my journal. Staying away from devices helps to reduce the risk of getting sucked into mindless scrolling.

Jan	Feb	Mar	Apr	May	Jun
Jul	Aug	Sep	Oct	(Nov)	Dec

Habit	1	2	3	4	5	6	7	8	9	10	11	12	13	14	15	16
Plan	✕	✕	✕	✕												
AM routine	✕	✕	✕													
PM routine	✕	✕	✕													
Protein	✕	✕	✕	✕	✕	✕	✕									

Habit	17	18	19	20	21	22	23	24	25	26	27	28	29	30	31
Plan															
AM routine															
PM routine															
Protein															

8 Week Strong for Life Program

In this chapter I'm going to help you map out the next 8 weeks so this can become part of your lifestyle long term.

Week 1: Orientation

Step 1:

Track what you eat for the next week (in an app like MyFitnessPal). This will give you an idea of where you are starting from. It will also help build more awareness about what you're eating.

Track your steps. If you have an iPhone, the health app will automatically track this for you. If not, download a step counting app. We want to note this data in order to figure out your average step count. We can then aim to improve it over the coming weeks.

Step 2:

Set your weekly floor goal. This is the minimum number of workouts you plan on doing every single week regardless of how busy life becomes. To work this out, think about what a hellish week would look like. This would be a week where everything goes wrong. We've all had them. Work is crazy, you're travelling or you're feeling tired and sick.

What can you still show up and do that week?

Many of you might reply: "4 x 45-minute sessions!" That's awesome, but I want you to remember to *under promise and over deliver*. If you're unsure, I'd recommend 2 x 15-minute sessions as your weekly floor.

The goal needs to be small, because I want you to create a habit of showing up *every single* week regardless of how you feel. In order to achieve this, it has to be easy.

Step 3:

Schedule your workouts into your calendar. I'd recommend slotting in two mornings if possible. You might choose 7am on Tuesday and Thursday as your workout times. I prefer working out in the morning because less things get in the way. When you put off your workout until the evening, many issues can crop up to distract you. We want to set times that you can do consistently each week over the coming year.

When you have set times, you don't need to think about it. You just execute it because it's 7am on Tuesday and that's when you work out.

> Weekly review:
>
> Rate your week out of 10 (10 being awesome, 1 being miserable).
>
> What went well this week?
>
> What can you improve upon for next week?
>
> Did you notice anything from logging your food intake?

Week 2: Planning

In week 2, set aside time to plan your week ahead. I would suggest doing this on the weekend. Then decide how many days of the week you can commit to planning daily and at what time. To increase your chances of success, try to implement your planning time into a habit you already have. For example, if you have coffee every morning at 8am, you might decide to schedule your planning session after your morning coffee.

Again, I recommend under-committing here. It might be a realistic goal to aim for a planning session on Monday, Tuesday and Wednesday.

Here's an example of how Week 2 might look:

- Sunday – Plan week – write down your MIT's (Most Important Tasks) and assign them to the relevant days of the week.
- Monday – Plan your day when you're having your morning coffee.

- Tuesday – 7am workout, followed by planning your day whilst drinking your morning coffee.
- Wednesday – Plan your day whilst drinking your morning coffee.
- Thursday – 7am workout
- Friday –
- Saturday –

If you stick to the above example, your week will be a success. Of course, if you want to make a greater commitment, you can. In fact, most of you probably will. The aim is to create long-term behavioural changes. It's easy to stick to something for 30 days, but it's a completely different story when it comes to 3 years.

The biggest trap is to over commit at the start. If you miss a workout in the first week, you'll assume you've failed and you'll end up quitting

Weekly review:
Rate your week out of 10 (10 being awesome, 1 being miserable).
What went well this week?

What can you improve on next week?

Did you succeed with your planning commitment?

How much planning do you want to do next week?

Week 3: AM/PM routines

In week 3, the aim is to continue your planning sessions and minimal workout commitments. At this stage, we also want to introduce AM & PM routines. As mentioned in an earlier chapter, sleep is the single greatest performance enhancer.

The goal is to adjust your AM and PM routines into realistic habits. A suggestion would be to follow the AM & PM routine listed below. Try it for three days out of the week, setting aside 10 minutes for the AM routine and 30 minutes for the PM wind down.

Suggestions for the AM routine using the **SAVERS** model:

- Silence – Sit and focus on your breath. I like Andrew Weil's 4/7/8 breathing technique. Inhale for 4,

hold for 7, exhale for 8. Repeat 3 times.
- **A**ffirmations – Repeat some motivational words.
- **V**isualisation – Visualise how you want the day to go.
- **E**xercise – Do some hip and shoulder mobility.
- **R**ead – Read a paragraph from a motivational book.
- **S**cribe – Write out your daily plan using the journaling questions:
  - o What 3 things would make today great? (Controllable activities eg. workout.)
  - o What am I grateful for?
  - o What are my MIT(s)?

You can pick one or two of these or do them all for 1-2 minutes each.

PM wind down options:

- Turn off electronics – phone, laptop, TV.
- Read some fiction.
- Brian dump/ journal:

- o What are my MIT(s) tomorrow?
- o Do I need to message anyone?
- o What 3 wins or awesome things happened today?
- o Where can I improve?
- o Who did I impact today?

Here's an example of how week 3 might look:

- Sunday – Plan week – write down all MIT's (Most Important Tasks) and schedule them to the days you plan on doing them. 30 min PM
- Monday – 10 min AM, plan day with morning coffee, 30 min PM
- Tuesday – 10 min AM, 7am workout, plan day with morning coffee, 30 min PM
- Wednesday – 10 min AM, plan day with morning coffee.
- Thursday – 7am workout.
- Friday –
- Saturday –

Weekly review:

Rate your week out of 10 (10 being awesome, 1 being miserable).

What went well this week?

What can you improve on next week?

Did you succeed with your planning & AM/PM commitment?

Did you feel any different with sleep or energy?

How much of each habit do you want to do next week?

Week 4: Protein

This week we are focusing on adding more protein into your diet. We are going to scale this habit like you've done each week with the other habits. You will also continue with your planning, and your AM/PM routines. Again, under-commit!

For the ease of this example, I'm going to assume you eat 3 meals a day. If you eat more or less, you can adjust accordingly. So, 3 meals daily x 7 days = 21 meals a week.

Out of 21 meals, try to commit to having more protein at a set number of them. On the low end I'd recommend 10, on the higher end, 15-18. So, let's say you commit to having protein in 10 meals this week.

It might be realistic to include protein in each of your 7 dinners and in 3 of your lunches – making a total of 10 meals.

How much should you eat?

As I covered in the nutrition chapter, take your weight number in lbs and convert it to grams to get your recommended amount. I weigh 175 lbs which means I should be aiming for 175 grams of protein each day.

To get the amount of food, I'll multiply this by 5 to get 875 grams of meat. To get the amount per meal, I'll divide it by 3 to give me 290 grams per meal.

If you weigh the same as me, you are aiming for 290 grams of meat/ fish/ poultry for 10 meals. Adjust this accordingly to fit your body weight.

Here's an example of how week 4 might look.

- Sunday – Plan week – write down all MIT's (Most Important Tasks) and schedule them to the days you plan on doing them. 30 min PM, Protein dinner.

- Monday – 10 min AM, plan day with morning coffee, 30 min PM, protein lunch & dinner.
- Tuesday – 10 min AM, 7am workout, plan day with morning coffee, 30 min PM. Protein lunch & dinner.
- Wednesday – 10 min AM, plan day with morning coffee. Protein lunch and dinner.
- Thursday – 7am workout, Protein dinner.
- Friday – Protein dinner.
- Saturday – Protein dinner.

Weekly review:

Rate your week out of 10 (10 being awesome, 1 being miserable).

What went well this week?

What can you improve on next week?

Did you succeed with your commitments?

If not, why were they challenging?

Did you feel any different with sleep & energy?

Which habit do you want to continue with next week?

Week 5: More steps (OTM's)

We're into month 2. I hope you are feeling better. Most importantly, I hope you feel this is manageable. I want this to feel like it's something you can continue in the long term. If you're struggling, it's time to scale things back. If it feels easy, you can adjust the dial and make things a bit more challenging.

This week the focus is on OTM's (Opportunities To Move). Awareness around lifestyle habits is the main thing I coach my clients on. If you're on autopilot mode, you will default to comfort. The modern world is set up for you to move as little as possible. This week we are focusing on changing that.

Whatever your average step count was in week one, this week we are focusing on adding an extra 1,000 steps a day. Walking more means you are sitting less. This leads to better mobility and less stiffness. The simple act of walking more is also clinically proven to improve lower back pain.

I also want you to audit your week. Where are you driving or sitting when you could be standing or walking? One of my clients parks her car further away from her kids' school and they walk the rest of the way. Instead of dealing with traffic and having difficulty parking close to the school, they enjoy fresh air and a walk together each morning.

Here are some other tips you can apply:

- Park further away from the store.
- Go for a 10-minute walk in the morning, after a meal and/or after you finish work. If you work from home, a walk can be a nice transition activity to end your workday and start your evening routine.
- For every 30 minutes of sitting, stand for 2 minutes. Set an alarm or timer and use this as a productivity block. I use the *Be Focused* app on my MacBook and do work blocks this way.

- Move between a standing desk, a sitting desk and ground sitting. This might not be realistic if you're in an office, but I strongly recommend this if you work from home. Moving between these positions will do wonders for your hips and lower back.
- Schedule in a longer walk for 45+ minutes 2-3 days a week.
- Take phone calls while you stand or walk.
- Do walking meetings and walk with a friend when you catch up.

Here's an example of how week 5 might look.

- Sunday – Plan week – write down all MIT's (Most Important Tasks) and schedule the days you plan on doing them. 30 min PM, Protein dinner. 45 min walk.
- Monday – 10 min AM, AM walk, plan day with morning coffee, 30 min PM, protein lunch & dinner.

- Tuesday – 10 min AM, 7am workout, plan day with morning coffee, 30 min PM. Protein lunch & dinner. 45 min walk.
- Wednesday – 10 min AM, AM walk, plan day with morning coffee. Protein lunch and dinner.
- Thursday – 7am workout, Protein dinner.
- Friday – AM walk, Protein dinner.
- Saturday – AM walk, Protein dinner.

Weekly review:

Rate your week out of 10 (10 being awesome, 1 being miserable).

What went well this week?

What can you improve on next week?

Did you succeed with your commitments?

If not, why were they challenging?

Did you feel any different with sleep & energy?

Which habits do you want to continue next week?

Week 6: Put your fork down

If you rush your meals, chances are, you're rushing other parts of your life. This week, we're focusing on slowing down when eating your meals. The simple act of putting your fork down between bites will help you get a better understanding of your hunger levels and reduce the likelihood of overeating.

It takes about 20 minutes for the signals from your stomach to reach your brain. If you hoover your food up in less than 5 minutes, it's easy to feel like you are still hungry and then overeat.

This is how to practice this food skill:

- Take a mouthful of food.
- Put down your fork.
- Chew your food at least 10 times.
- Swallow.
- Take a deep breath.
- Repeat.

If you are a fast eater (like me) this will slow you down a lot. You'll also enjoy your food a lot more and reduce the likelihood of overeating.

Now it's time to decide how many meals you want to practice this skill. Again, assuming you eat 21 times a week (3 times a day X 7 days), decide on a number. I would recommend starting with 7 times a week for this one. Dinner tends to work best for people as breakfast and lunch are often rushed.

Here's an example of how week 6 might look.

- Sunday – plan week – write down all MIT's (Most Important tasks) and schedule them to the days you plan on doing them. 30 min PM, Protein dinner (fork down). 45 min walk.
- Monday – 10 min AM, AM walk, plan day with morning coffee, 30 min PM, protein lunch & dinner (fork down).
- Tuesday – 10 min AM, 7am workout, plan day with morning coffee, 30 min PM. Protein lunch & dinner (fork down). 45 min walk.

- Wednesday – 10 min AM, AM walk, plan day with morning coffee. Protein lunch and dinner (fork down).
- Thursday – 7am workout, Protein dinner (fork down).
- Friday – AM walk, Protein dinner (fork down).
- Saturday – AM walk, Protein dinner (fork down).

Weekly review:

Rate your week out of 10 (10 being awesome, 1 being miserable).

What went well this week?

What can you improve on next week?

Did you succeed with your commitments?

If not, why were they challenging?

Did you feel any different with sleep & energy?

Which habits do you want to continue next week?

Week 7: Plan & prep your meals

This week I'm going to teach you how to become a meal prep ninja. It needs to be easy if you're going to do this long term. Not having healthy food in the fridge is the biggest reason why most people opt for take-out or junk food.

If your fridge is stocked up with tasty food, your chances of eating well are almost guaranteed. The first step is to create a meal plan for the week and month ahead. The next step is to prepare the meals. Below is the simple system I use which only takes ten minutes. I teach my clients this system to help them create meals for four weeks.

Days	Protein	Cuisine	Recipe
Monday	Poultry	Western	Roast chicken
Tuesday	Beef	Mexican	Beef tacos
Wednesday	Lentils/Beans	French	French lentils
Thursday	Pork	USA	Slow cooked pulled pork
Friday	Fish	Thai	Tom Yum Soup
Saturday	Veg	Mediterranean	Halloumi salad
Sunday	Lamb	Western	Slow cooked lamb shank

In the above grid, I organise daily meals according to protein sources, types of cuisine and the specific recipe. You can adapt this to suit your preferences as this is just a template. However, focusing on which protein you'll have as your meal base will ensure you'll eat meals that are rich in protein. It will also help to keep things simple.

This starts to make even more sense when we look at how we can incorporate lots of variety without changing the base ingredients. In the image below, I show several examples of beef mince recipes for each week of the month. The Mexican style meal is beef tacos, the Italian cuisine is beef Bolognese, the Thai style is Pad Kra Pao and another Italian dish is beef meatballs. The only changes with these recipes are the spices. You can use the same base ingredients for all of these recipes – beef mince, garlic, onions, and red peppers.

For the Mexican tacos you can use a taco mix or make your own. For the Bolognese and meatballs, you can use tinned tomatoes, basil and oregano. For the Pad Kra

Pao, you can use oyster, fish and soy sauce along with basil or Thai holy basil.

After that, it's just a case of deciding what carbohydrate you want to add. For the tacos, you could use corn or wheat tortillas. Alternatively, you could use iceberg lettuce for a low carb option. For the Italian dishes, you could use pasta or spaghetti. For a low carb option, you could use Zucchini noodles. For the Pad Kra Pao, you could use rice or, for the lower carb option; cauliflower rice.

Week 1	Cuisine	Recipe	Week 2	Cuisine	Recipe
Beef	Mexican	Beef tacos	Beef	Italian	Bolognese
Week 3	Cuisine	Recipe	Week 4	Cuisine	Recipe
Beef	Thai	Pad Krapao	Beef	Italian	Meatballs

To give you a completely new cuisine, you can simply change the spices you use. Of course, you don't need to have as much variety. Personally, I stick to the same two or three cuisines and eat similar stuff each week. On the other hand, my brother loves variety and wants a different style of food at every meal. Find out what suits you and your household the best.

Another tip is to batch cook. Instead of cooking dinner for 4 people (1 portion each), cook enough for 12 or 16 people (3-4 portions each). You can then freeze the leftovers. After a few weeks of doing this, you'll have a freezer full of meals.

Two habits to focus on this week are planning meals and batch cooking meals. You can adapt this to suit your lifestyle – either planning meals for one month or scaling down to planning meals for one week. You could also batch cook meals for one week or just double the portions each time you cook and freeze the rest.

Here's an example of how week 7 might look:

- Sunday – Plan week – write down all MIT's (Most Important Tasks) and schedule the days you plan on doing them. Plan meals for next week. 30 min PM, Protein dinner (fork down) – cook enough for 4 meals. 45 min walk.
- Monday – 10 min AM, AM walk, plan day with morning coffee, 30

min PM, protein lunch & dinner (fork down).

- Tuesday – 10 min AM, workout at 7am, plan day with morning coffee, 30 min PM. Protein lunch & dinner (fork down). 45 min walk.
- Wednesday – 10 min AM, AM walk, plan day with morning coffee. Protein lunch and dinner (fork down) cook enough for 4 meals.
- Thursday – workout at 7am, Protein dinner (fork down).
- Friday – AM walk, Protein dinner (fork down).
- Saturday – AM walk, Protein dinner (fork down).

Weekly review:

Rate your week out of 10 (10 being awesome, 1 being miserable).

What went well this week?

What can you improve next week?

Did you succeed with your commitments?

If not, why were they challenging?

Did you feel any different with sleep & energy?

How much of each habit do you want to do next week?

Week 8: Review of program to date and plan for next month.

Welcome to week 8. This is the final week of the program, but only the beginning of your journey. I hope you found the last 7 weeks valuable and feel that you can sustain these habits. Now it's time to review what went well for you and what you want to focus on going forward.

Step 1:

Track your food and steps for the next week. Compare them to what you tracked in week 1. Have they improved?

Step 2:

Review how your workout schedule went. Did the times you allocated work? If so, do you want to add more sessions?

Step 3:

Focus on one habit.

I don't think it's necessary to continue with everything we've covered. This week, I want you to reflect on how the last 7 weeks have gone and pick one habit that you want to focus on.

Once you decide the habit you want to focus on, make the commitment a little harder than you had been doing. If you are focusing on the AM/PM routines and you tried a 10-minute AM routine and 30-minute PM routine for 3 days you can try adding more days to these habits.

For example: AM routine for 30 minutes x 5 days, PM routine for 60 minutes x 5 days.

Moving forwards, each week you can reflect on how the previous week has gone and what area you want to focus on. Here are some tips depending on your goal.

Goal – Fitness, mobility improvements, pain reduction.

Habits – OTMs, planning, more workout frequency.

Goal – body composition, fat loss, energy.

Habits – meal prep, protein, planning, AM/PM routines, fork down.

Goal – longevity

Habits – AM/PM routine, OTMs, fork down.

Thank You

If you made it this far, I appreciate you taking time out of your schedule and investing in your health.

I wanted this book to be a simple, straightforward guide that you could read in one sitting; a book that can give you clarity on training and nutrition. This stuff is simple to understand, but not easy to integrate.

These systems and techniques took me sixteen years to develop, not only on myself, but on my clients. It's a collection of tips and advice I have gathered from mentors over the years. It's a book I wish someone handed to me at the beginning of my training journey. I hope it will save you a lot of the pain and mistakes I made when I first started out.

If you like this approach, but feel you need accountability to execute it, please click the link below to learn more about my coaching program. Reading and implementing are two very different things
www.conorosheafitness.com/online-coaching.html

Lastly, if you found this book helpful, please share it with a friend and leave a review so I can reach more people.

Thanks,
Conor O' Shea

About the Author

Conor O'Shea has been coaching since 2011.

Having spent his childhood playing Gaelic games, he found himself riddled with injuries in his early 20's. After studying sport science and trying different bodybuilding workouts, he set out on a path to fix his injuries.

He spent two years in Asia, practising and teaching Hatha and Ashtanga yoga. He also spent six years in Australia running an in-person coaching business and doing numerous mentorships with some of the top coaches in Australia.

In 2016, he qualified as a GMB Fitness trainer. This gave him a framework which combined the knowledge he had acquired from Sport and Exercise Science, Yoga and strength and conditioning into a system that worked well for rehabbing his own body and his clients.

He focuses on a holistic approach with clients, meeting them where they're at and helping them reach their goals in a sustainable way.

He now runs his business 100% remotely, serving clients all over the world.

The Strong for Life Podcast

Conor O'Shea hosts the Strong for Life podcast where he interviews the best minds in the health and fitness industry.

He also interviews clients who have followed his coaching program: *The Strong For Life Blueprint.*

You can listen to the podcast here: www.conorosheafitness.com/about.html or on Spotify or Apple

Printed in Great Britain
by Amazon